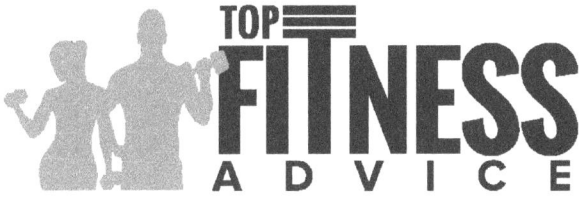

TOP FITNESS ADVICE

DETOX

5-Day Weight Loss Cleanse & Detox Diet To Get Healthy And Boost Your Metabolism (With Juicing Meal Plan + Smoothie Recipes)

Kayla Bates

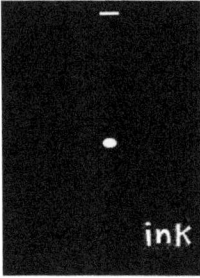

Disclaimer

This book provides wellness management information in an informative and educational manner only, with information that is general in nature and that is not specific to you, the reader. The contents of this book are intended to assist you and other readers in your personal wellness efforts. Consult your physician regarding the applicability of any information provided in this book to you.

Nothing in this book should be construed as personal advice or diagnosis, and must not be used in this manner. The information provided about conditions is general in nature. This information does not cover all possible uses, actions, precautions, side-effects, or interactions of medicines, or medical procedures. The information in this book should not be considered as complete and does not cover all diseases, ailments, physical conditions, or their treatment.

You should consult with your physician before beginning any exercise, weight loss, or health care program. This book should not be used in place of a call or visit to a competent health-care professional. You should consult a health care professional before adopting any of the suggestions in this book or before drawing inferences from it.

Any decision regarding treatment and medication for your condition should be made with the advice and consultation of a qualified health care professional. If you have, or suspect you have, a health-care problem, then you should immediately contact a qualified health care professional for treatment.

No Warranties: The author and publisher don't guarantee or warrant the quality, accuracy, completeness, timeliness, appropriateness or suitability of the information in this book, or of any product or services referenced in this book.

The information in this book is provided on an "as is" basis and the author and publisher make no representations or warranties of any kind with respect to this information. This book may contain inaccuracies, typographical errors, or other errors.

Table of Contents

Would you prefer to listen to my book, rather than read it?

Download the audiobook version for free!

If you go to the special link below and sign up to Audible as a new customer, you can get the audiobook version of my book completely free.

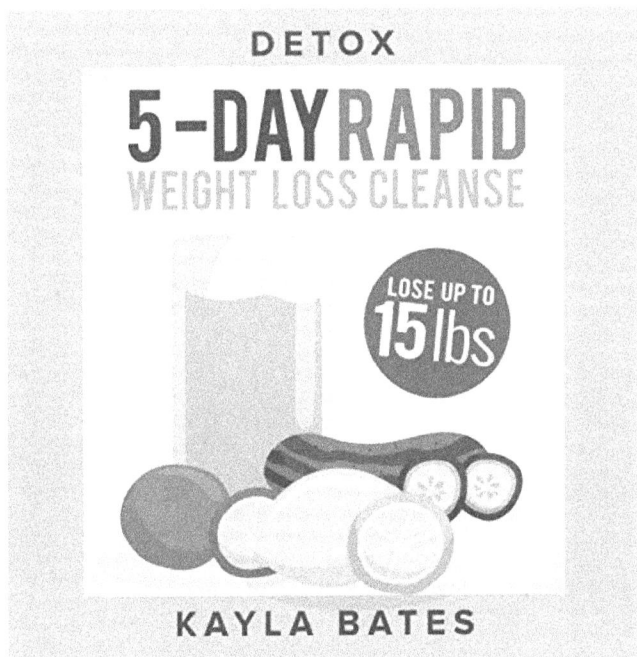

Go here to get your audiobook version for free:

TopFitnessAdvice.com/go/Detox5Day

Who is this book for?

Have you tried every diet plan out there, every piece of equipment available for losing weight and keeping it off, only to see you're your stubborn belly fat and numbers on the scale refuse to budge?

Do you feel sluggish and fatigued at the same time, no matter what you eat and what weight loss plan you try?

If so, you may simply need to detoxify! When the body holds toxins without filtering them out and getting rid of them as it should, those toxins can make it difficult to burn fat and lose weight, and may make you feel tired and rundown.

Detoxifying doesn't mean taking harsh powders that upset your system and actually remove healthy and helpful bacteria from your digestive tract.

Instead, it means making a few simple choices for how you eat, and then giving your body a break from toxins and hurtful substances for a few days, while it's natural filters catch up. This can help you to finally lose that extra weight and get back the energy you need every single day.

Detoxifying is easy and can be done by anyone, and can help you lose up to 15 pounds in just 5 days, while protecting your health and restoring your body to overall good health.

What will this book teach you?

Your body takes in a number of toxins through what you eat every single day, and these needs to be trapped and then flushed out of your system regularly.

Your body has natural ways of doing this, as most toxins you ingest are caught in the liver and then flushed out as bile or secreted through your urine.

Your body also breathes in toxins every single day, no matter where you live or your everyday schedule; you're always breathing in pollution, chemicals, dust, and irritants like animal hair and dander, as well as dead skin cells.

These things are simply in the air around you, even if you don't smoke, don't have a pet, keep your home very dust free, and have filters and ventilation in the home.

These irritants are caught in the lungs and then filtered through the bloodstream and out of the body. Antioxidants also fight off these toxins; these are agents that fight what are called free radicals, or outside toxins like pollution and cigarette smoke.

Antioxidants are made up of vitamins, trace minerals, and other such nutrients that you get in foods and beverages like fresh fruit, green vegetables, and green tea.

While the body has this natural way of getting rid of toxins, you don't want to always rely on its systems or just the liver and lungs alone to get this done for you.

The liver can begin to break down over time, as do the lungs, and having too many toxins in your system can overwhelm these organs so that those toxins begin to build up and then may get absorbed by your system rather than being flushed out properly.

The right diet and some healthier lifestyle choices can mean getting rid of these toxins more easily and more often, so that they don't build up in your system and cause damage to healthy cells.

This book will tell you how to get rid of these toxins in a healthy, safe way, and how to avoid that dangerous buildup of toxins that can destroy your health, cause fatigue, and get in the way of your weight loss goals.

The Most Common Toxins You Put in Your Body

To better understand how to get rid of toxins in the body, you want to consider the most common toxins that wind up there in the first place, as some may surprise you.

This can also help you to see the importance of making certain changes in order to keep out those toxins or reduce your intake of them, rather than just assuming you can flush them out with dietary changes.

Caffeine

Caffeine in small doses may be easy for your body to metabolize and then flush out of your system, but far too many people have large amounts of caffeine throughout the day, so that this toxin builds up very easily.

You may not realize the amount of caffeine you're ingesting every day, as you may not realize the many foods and beverages that contain caffeine.

Coffee, tea, and cola are obvious culprits, but many other sodas, energy drinks, and even some brands of bottled water will have caffeine added to them. Chocolate also contains caffeine, as do many protein bars and shakes, and of course candy bars with chocolate.

Certain yogurt brands and breakfast bars in particular may also have added caffeine, as these are typically eaten in the morning for breakfast.

Caffeine stimulates the adrenaline glands, causing the body to produce adrenaline, which is how it gives you that immediate boost of energy.

However, having too much caffeine, too often, can easily wear out those adrenaline glands so that they don't produce as much adrenaline as quickly or as effectively as they once did.

In turn, they may cause your body to crave even more caffeine so that they can produce adrenaline more easily. This toxin can then build up in the liver and in the bloodstream.

Diet soda

Diet sodas deserves a mention apart from the caffeine it contains, as the artificial sweeteners in diet soda contain the same chemicals as embalming fluid and other harmful substances.

Many people switch to diet soda when they want to trim their waistline or watch their sugar intake, but if you're concerned about toxins, this is not the right choice for your diet!

The chemicals that make up soda as well as those that create the sweet taste of diet soda can easily build up in your liver and cause a toxic overload.

Carbs, and especially bread

Wheat is very healthy in that it has a large amount of fiber, which your body needs for proper digestion and to absorb the vitamins and trace minerals of other foods.

However, there are also toxins in wheat that can easily build up in your system when you have a lot of bread and other foods made from wheat.

Many people have more bread than they realize, as it's a staple for lunchtime sandwiches as well as a quick filler for breakfast and dinnertime.

A few pieces of toast or bread slices can fill in the gaps of your meals and make you feel full, so it's not unusual for people to eat large amounts of bread as well as rolls, bagels, muffins, and other foods containing wheat throughout their day.

Canned foods

Canned foods contain an enormous amount of preservatives, in order to keep foods edible while in a can and not a refrigerator!

These preservatives are very toxic to your system and don't get broken down into your digestive system along with other foods. In turn, they build up along the liver and even in the digestive system itself.

Some studies suggest that preservatives used for canned foods are so toxic that they may cause hyperactivity and other behavior disorders in children, as well as certain forms of cancer.

While more studies need to be done, it's obvious that these chemicals are not good for you and can easily be considered toxic and dangerous!

Processed meats

Processed meats are those that have ingredients added to them, rather than being plain cuts of meat. This would include bacon, ham, lunchmeat, jerky, any type of canned meat such as Spam, and the like.

The chemicals used in the processing, as well as the large amounts of sodium, can mean a quick buildup of toxins in your system.

Salt or sodium can also hold water so that your body cannot easily flush out any toxins or harmful agents. These meats also typically have a very high fat content, and body fat may hold toxins in your system so that they build up and affect all your cells and tissue.

Cheese, Yogurt

The processing that goes into making cheese and yogurt means that bacteria is created in these foods. This bacteria is harmless and even beneficial in small amounts; however, as with caffeine and so many other toxins, it's easy to overlook how much of this type of food you're getting in your everyday diet.

You might have yogurt for breakfast, cheese on your sandwich or salad for lunch, and then more cheese on your potatoes or veggies at dinnertime. Another yogurt cup might be your convenient midnight snack before bedtime.

At the end of the day, you've added quite a bit of bacteria to your system and this could be very harmful.

Fried foods

Light oils that are easy to digest, such as olive oil or avocado oil, can be very good for you when you use them on a salad or to toss with vegetables.

However, when you heat up oils, you cause a chemical reaction that destabilizes these oil molecules, creating damaging free radicals that attack healthy cells in your body.

The most damaging type of oil is hydrogenated or partially hydrogenated; this is the term used when hydrogen is introduced into the oil in order to keep it stable during the shipping and storage process, such as needed for food service businesses.

The more of these oils you have, and the more fried foods you have in general, the more toxins that build up in your body.

Alcohol

It may not be surprising to learn that alcohol contains many toxins that can be very damaging to your liver, when consumed in large amounts. Those toxins deplete your body of vitamin B, which can lead to fatigue. Those toxins also interfere with memory, which is why you may not be able to remember a night of binge drinking!

Alcohol causes you to lose hydration, which is why you develop a headache or hangover the next day; your body needs this hydration to flush toxins out of your system.

The toxins in alcohol are so strong that many forms of liver disease are associated with overdrinking, as these toxins overload the liver and cause early breakdown.

Saturated fats

Saturated fats get trapped in your bloodstream since the body cannot break them down and digest them very easily. They then trap toxins and can cause damage to healthy cells, as they are delivered by the blood to every part of the body.

Saturated fats include butter and any fats from dairy products, as well as vegetable oil and coconut oil and fats from meat products including beef fat and the skin of chicken.

Cigarette smoke

Cigarette smoke may not be a surprise when it comes to toxins in the body, but keep in mind that filtered cigarettes, "light" cigarettes, and even vapor cigarettes can have lots of toxins that wind up in your lungs.

Filters in cigarettes only filter out a small number of toxins, and a "light" cigarette doesn't mean it's without tar, nicotine, and other positions.

Vapor cigarettes still involve breathing in irritating and damaging smoke, even though you're not taking in nicotine. Secondhand smoke can also be very damaging and toxic.

Volatile organic compounds

Volatile organic compounds or VOCs are very toxic to the body and yet, we are surrounded by them every day, and often introduce them to our systems without thinking about it.

These are found in fumes from cleaning solutions, as well as paint, solvents, and the like, you are always exposing yourself to these harmful toxins. You can easily absorb them through your skin, through the fumes you breathe in, and even through your digestive system as they get into your throat.

Are You ALWAYS Hungry When You Try to Lose Weight?

Discover How to STOP Starving Yourself & Lose Weight FASTER By Eating MORE Food!

For this month only, you can get Kayla's best-selling & most popular book absolutely free – *The Ultimate Guide to Healthy Eating & Losing Weight Without Starving Yourself!*

Get Your FREE Copy Here:

TopFitnessAdvice.com/Book

Discover how you can **start eating MORE food** and see weight loss results faster than ever before. Learn about the 10 most powerful fat-burning foods and how they boost the rate that your body burns fat. And last but not least, finally put an end to your emotional or "bored" eating habits. With this book, readers were able to significantly improve their weight loss results. So, it's highly recommended that you get this book, especially while it's free!

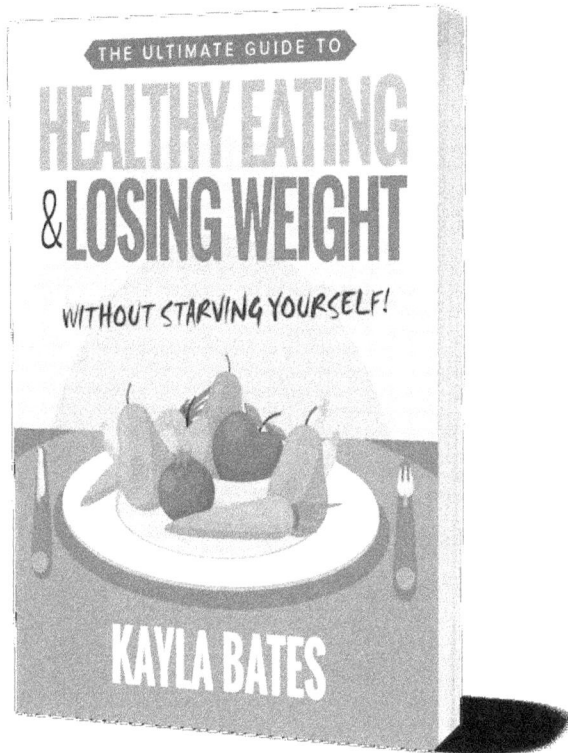

Get Your FREE Copy Here:

TopFitnessAdvice.com/Book

Chapter 1

How the Liver Works to Detoxify Your Body

The liver will trap and clear out toxins you ingest through eating and drinking. The liver helps to detoxify the body in a number of ways; consider them here.

Filtering

After eating, food particles are sent through the liver so that they can be broken down and filtered even further. The liver will trap harmful enzymes that don't belong in your bloodstream and then secrete them as bile back into your digestive system so they can be eliminated, or will mix them with uric acid so you can release them through your urine.

Ammonia, created and released when you eat protein, is also then converted to uric acid and expelled.

Another way that the liver filters toxins is by using a concentration of oxygen and enzymes to actually burn away those toxins so they aren't absorbed into your system. Any other toxins it cannot break down are then carried to the small intestine or the kidneys, to be expelled as waste.

Hormones and immune system

Your immune system plays a vital role in your overall toxicity levels; when the immune system is weak, it does not produce enough red blood and white blood cells to fight off infection, viruses, and the like, and to repair and rebuild damaged tissue.

A weakened immune system can then also mean that your body is allowing these toxins to build up in the system, and in the bloodstream in particular.

The liver protects your immune system first by regulating certain hormones in the body.

The liver will break down stress hormones such as cortisol, insulin, and adrenaline, and then clear excess amounts from the bloodstream.

Too much of any of these hormones in your system and your immune system becomes weak, and your body is not able to filter out toxins as it should.

The liver also converts vitamin D, creating it from the chemical reaction when sunlight hits your skin; vitamin D is very important for your overall health and immunity. Without sufficient levels of this vitamin, you may become fatigued and even depressed, as your immune system gets weakened.

Chapter 2

How the Lungs Detoxify the Body

Lungs are an important detoxifying part of the body; they don't just bring in fresh air and expel bad air, but will also work to trap irritants that you breathe in or that comes into your system because of coming into contact with your skin.

Consider how the lungs work to detoxify the body as you can then better understand how to support them and strengthen them, just as you do your liver.

When your body collects certain toxins or these get absorbed into the body through your skin, throat, and the like, they are often collected by the blood as it makes its way around the body. The blood then travels through the mucus lining of the lungs; this mucus traps those antigens and toxins so they can be expelled when you exhale. This keeps them from re-circulating through the body.

Lungs also bolster your immune system by bringing in fresh oxygen that it filters through that mucus as well. This captures some of the pollutants and irritants in the air around you, so that those harmful toxins don't make their way to your body's cells by way of the bloodstream.

This fresh oxygen works as a healing agent; an oxygen molecule is delivered to all the cells of the body by way of the bloodstream, and that oxygen then repairs and restores that cell.

This strengthens your immune system and helps the body get rid of harmful toxins and irritants, while also helping organs like the liver repair and rebuild itself so it, too, can continue to filter toxins out of the body.

I hope that you are enjoying this book so far, and if you could spare 30 seconds, I would greatly appreciate you leaving a review on Amazon.com.

Chapter 3

Protecting and Strengthening the Liver

Because the liver plays such a vital role in detoxifying the body, you want to ensure you're doing everything you can to protect and strengthen this vital organ.

Note a few tips on how to do this, before we talk about ways to support it with a detoxifying program you follow on your own.

Reduce Alcohol Consumption

If alcohol is one of the main causes of toxins building up in your liver and cause the most damage to your liver, then of course you should consider reducing your consumption as needed.

It can be good to be honest with yourself about how much you drink and how often; remember, this is for your overall health.

If you drink every day, switch to other beverages that you consider an indulgence but which don't have those toxins, such as fresh fruit juice mixed with seltzer water for a nice kick.

Opt for nonalcoholic drinks and beers. Mix up fresh smoothies to take the place of daiquiris and margaritas. You can also limit yourself to just having a limited number of drinks on a Saturday night versus drinking every night, or whatever else you need to do to cut back to a healthy amount.

Reduce Fatty Foods

Saturated fats can surround the liver and get in the way of its filtering process, and also trap toxins in your bloodstream and around other organs. The liver then needs to work harder to filter out toxins in your system.

Reducing fatty foods isn't always as easy as you might think, as there are many foods that contain added fat in order to enhance their flavor. This might include canned soups, stews, and chili.

Remember, too, that snack foods like pretzels are actually fried rather than baked, as are potato chips, cheese puffs, and other similar foods.

Lubricating the Liver

One of the best ways you can keep the liver healthy is by keeping it lubricated.

All the organs and muscles of the body need proper hydration and moisture or lubrication to function; this will help keep the liver supple and strong so it can keep filtering out toxins.

Lubricating the liver means having lots of healthy fats and oils in your system; not saturated fats, as mentioned above, but lighter fats like olive oil, avocado oil, and oil from walnuts. These fats are easy for your body to break down and absorb and will help keep the liver strong.

Drinking Water

Because the liver needs to stay supple to work as an organ, drinking water is also very necessary. This will help break down those toxins and keep them flowing to the digestive tract so the liver doesn't need to work as hard to capture and filter them.

Water also keeps the cells and tissues of the liver itself healthy and strong, so it works as a better filter overall.

Water is needed by all cells of the body to repair and restore themselves, so you need to stay hydrated so the liver can repair itself from any damage it suffers over the years.

Eliminating

The liver works to filter toxins and capture them, and then pass them along the digestive tract where they are excreted through urine or your elimination.

Because of this, it's vital that you have regular, healthy elimination, so that those toxins don't build up in the system and cause the liver to work overtime.

If you're dehydrated, you won't be able to urinate as often as you should; if you suffer from regular constipation and other bowel issues, this too can interfere with proper elimination.

Adding fiber to your diet and reducing your caffeine intake can help with proper elimination so that your digestive system and, in turn, your liver both stay healthy.

Because the foods you eat are so important to detoxifying the liver and your body overall, let's look at which foods you'll want to add to your diet, or increase your intake of, in order to improve your liver's health and function and to help detox your system.

Chapter 4

The Right Foods to Detoxify the Liver

Certain foods can help the liver function better and break down harmful enzymes and other toxins so that they can be more easily absorbed and expelled by the digestive system.

Certain foods can also nourish the liver and help it to stay strong and healthy so it can more readily rebuild its own tissue and cells.

Consider a list of foods you want to increase in your everyday diet in order to strengthen the liver and support its overall function of detoxifying your body.

Leafy Green Veggies

Leafy green veggies are chockfull of antioxidants that help to break down toxins that are trapped around the liver, so they can be more easily absorbed into the digestive system.

They also neutralize heavy metals, meaning lead, nickel, and the like. This can keep them from entering the bloodstream and potentially poisoning your blood; even if this doesn't become life-threatening, a buildup of heavy metals and their poisons can mean damage to all cells and tissues of the body.

Note, it's good to get a variety of leafy greens so you enjoy the benefits of various antioxidants. Mix some dandelion greens, mustard greens, chicory, and a variety of romaine lettuces into your salad, or add a bunch of these greens to a smoothie or protein shake, as the other ingredients will mask the flavor.

Green Tea

Like green veggies, green tea has plenty of antioxidants that bolster your immune system and help to detoxify the liver.

If you add a bit of honey to sweeten it, this can help to coat your digestive system so that food moves along more easily and you're less prone to constipation; this will also help keep your liver healthy and strong.

You might also add a bit of lemon or even some cherry juice to cut down the flavor of green tea if it's a bit strong for you.

Honey

As said above, honey can coat the digestive tract so that foods can more easily move through your intestines and so that you have easier elimination.

Honey also has a lot of protein so that it can build strong muscles; the digestive system involves a series of muscles that work to move food and waste through the digestive tract.

Strengthening these muscles can mean better digestion and elimination, and less work for the liver overall.

Garlic

The pungent flavor of garlic is caused by its chemical properties, and these chemicals help the liver produce enzymes that break down toxins more readily.

You don't need a lot of garlic to enjoy its detoxifying benefits; add just a little bit to tomato sauces for your pasta dishes or to a beef dish, or roast garlic cloves to reduce the flavor while still enjoying the cleansing effect of this pungent bulb.

Grapefruit

The high acidic content of grapefruit may make it a bit pungent for your taste buds, but this type of acid is very healthy for your system and helps to break down toxins and cleanse the liver.

Grapefruit is also very high in vitamin C and other antioxidants that keep your immune system healthy.

If grapefruit juice is too tart, cut it with some water or add a bit of cherry juice to sweeten the taste.

Apples

The pectin in apples helps to cleanse the liver and rid the body of toxins.

Apples are also very high in fiber and moisture content, so they can more readily break down other foods you eat so these can move through your digestive system easily, meaning that your liver will need to flush out fewer toxins that get trapped in your system.

Apples make for a great snack on their own but you can also add them to your diet in a variety of ways.

Apple chunks are great in your morning oatmeal, or you might bake apples with a little bit of cinnamon for a warm dessert.

You can also use your own food processor to make homemade applesauce without harmful preservatives; heat this and add some ice cream for another simple and healthy dessert, or have it on its own with just a touch of cinnamon.

Cabbage

Cabbage contains a nutrient that helps the liver to produce an enzyme it needs to flush out toxins and do its job more efficiently.

While plain cabbage itself can be a bit bland, you might add more to your diet by mixing some fine shreds to your green salad or adding them to a sandwich.

Cabbage soup is also very filling, very high in fiber, and very low in calories, making it an all-around healthy choice.

Walnuts

The amino acids in walnuts in particular help the liver to function optimally.

Walnuts also have a natural oil that lubricates your insides and helps toxins move quickly through the system.

If you don't like plain walnuts, chop them and add them to salads or a smoothie, or to your ice cream desserts.

Once again, thank you for reading this book, and I hope you're getting a lot of valuable information. I would greatly appreciate it if you could take 30 seconds to leave me a review for this book on Amazon.com.

Chapter 5

What Is Meant By "Clean Eating" and How it Can Help You Detoxify

When researching how to detoxify your body, you may see many experts recommend "clean eating."

What is this, and how does it work to remove toxins from your system?

What Is Meant By Clean Eating

Clean eating doesn't mean taking away certain foods or watching how many calories you ingest; instead, it concentrates on the path that foods take from their origin to your stomach. This would include how the food is grown or harvested, how it is processed, and how it is prepared.

Consider some basic principles of clean eating and what this means. When you eat clean, you don't necessarily need to give up beef, but you should buy beef from grain-fed or grass-fed cows that are never given artificial hormones and steroids.

Meat and eggs should come from free-range chickens who are also raised without growth hormones or steroids.

Processing foods is very common, as preservatives and other materials are added to them so they stay fresh while being transported to stores and while on the shelves.

Clean eating would include eating as few of these processed foods as possible, and then substituting fresh foods and ingredients, even if it means making certain foods from scratch.

For instance, rather than buying canned soup loaded with preservatives as well as sugars and oils, you would buy fresh vegetables and meats and make soup from scratch when following a clean eating plan.

Processing also refers to changing the nature of foods and foodstuffs; as an example, wheat is processed so that the bran and wheat germ are removed, creating white flour, which has very few nutrients left over.

Tomatoes may be boiled to remove the skins so just the insides are used to create certain canned or jarred sauces, as skins may not be as flavorful as the inside "meat."

However, this also eliminates a lot of the fiber and many of the healthy vitamins and trace minerals in tomatoes.

What Clean Eating Doesn't Include

Some people are under the mistaken belief that clean eating means eating foods in their raw state.

It is true that overcooking foods and boiling them can eliminate some of their nutrients and lower their nutritional value, but cooking foods can also kill bacteria and toxins that would otherwise wind up in your body.

Cooking also creates a chemical reaction in food that is not always damaging or dangerous, but simply changes foods from one state to another; for example, mixing flour, sugar, water, oil, and other ingredients and then cooking them together allows them to coagulate and form bread. This isn't dangerous or unhealthy, and isn't contrary to a clean eating plan.

Cleaning eating plans may actually include many cooked and baked foods, as long as the foods themselves stay as close to their natural state as possible before they're cooked.

Clean eating also doesn't mean giving up ingredients or foodstuffs like sugar; in small amounts, sugar can be metabolized by your body and doesn't pose any harm.

Salt and other such flavorings, alcohol, and foodstuffs like these are usually dangerous to your health only when consumed in large amounts.

You can have small amounts of foods that you might consider to be unhealthy and still eat clean, including sugar, salt, alcohol, oil, beef, and the like.

How Clean Eating Helps With Detoxifying

There are a few ways that this type of clean eating can help with detoxifying your body.

One is that you are avoiding added toxins by not ingesting the chemicals that are used in food processing and as preservatives.

The fewer toxins you ingest, the fewer that may get caught in your system and that can't be filtered through the liver.

Also, when you follow a clean eating plan, you are getting more nutrients from foods that can help your liver to work better and more effectively.

If you don't ingest canned foods that have been processed and have had their nutrients stripped away from them, but eat more fresh foods or use fresh ingredients in your cooking, you will be getting more essential vitamins, trace minerals, amino acids, and other healthy nutrients.

These will strengthen your immunity, improve your blood circulation, help your body build red and white blood cells, and help the liver to repair and restore itself as needed.

While you may not be able to follow a clean eating plan completely, it's good to think of how many ways you can incorporate it into your daily diet.

For example, forego canned soups, stews, chili, and other such foods, and make these from scratch.

Stop eating boxed cereal, which is usually made with bleached and processed grains along with added chemicals, and have oatmeal, protein shakes, smoothies, or trail mix for breakfast.

You might also check if there is a farmer's market near your home where you can buy meat, dairy products, and other such foods from local farms that don't use steroids and growth hormones for their animals. You will also avoid all the preservatives used for such items when they are on supermarket shelves.

Enjoying this book?

Check out my other best sellers!

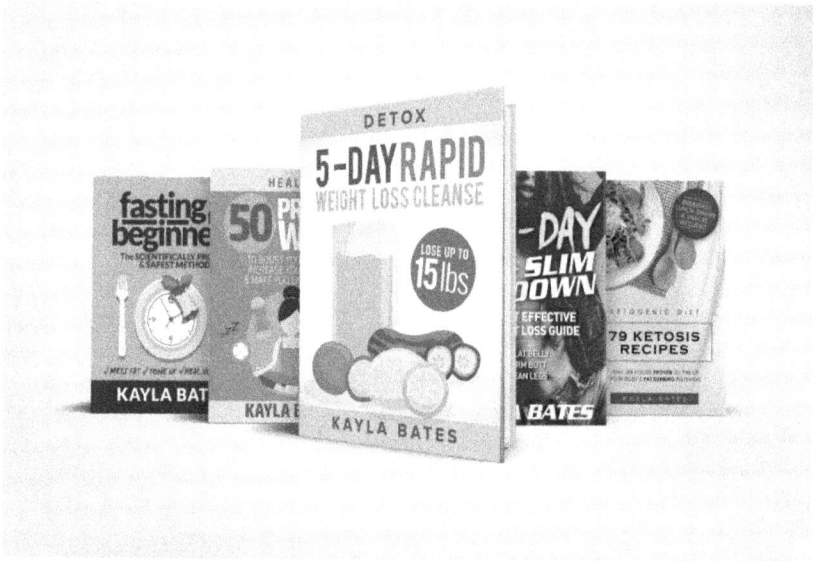

Get your next book on sale here:

TopFitnessAdvice.com/go/Kayla

Chapter 6

Fasting for Detoxifying

Fasting doesn't always necessarily mean going without food completely for long periods of time; a person might fast, meaning go without eating, for just a short time, and may also have a limited number of calories or foodstuffs during a fast.

Fasting can help your body to detoxify, as you're giving it a "break" from ingesting toxins altogether.

However, you don't want to think that you should just stop eating and especially should you stop drinking anything and everything altogether, assuming this is how to best help your system.

To understand how fasting can help with detoxifying, let's first talk about some ways that a person might hold or observe a fast, and some details involved in how to do this safely.

How To Safely Observe A Fast Cycle

To hold or observe a fast doesn't necessarily mean to go without any foods or anything to drink, as said above.

Instead, a person might simply severely limit their calorie intake for a certain amount of time.

For example, you might have a fast where you have no more than 500 calories in a 24-hour period. This is a little less than

1/4 the number of calories you might consume on average in that same time period.

You might spread out those calories over that 24-hour period, having a few calories for breakfast, lunch, and dinner, and then one or two very light snacks during the day as well.

You might also safely fast by alternating periods of fasting with periods of eating while still restricting your calories. For example, you might start a day with a 500-calorie breakfast and then fast for the next 24 hours, not eating until breakfast the next day.

You might do the same again on the second day, or may have a regular day of eating on the second day, then only a 500-calorie breakfast on the third day, and continue to rotate your schedule this way.

Another simple way to fast is to have a 12-hour observation; this would include a restricted calorie breakfast, perhaps no more than 300 calories, and then not eat for another 12 hours, allowing yourself a very light meal or snack at that 12-hour point, then going another 12 hours without eating.

During a fast, you also want to ensure that you drink plenty of water to stay hydrated and help your body break down the toxins that have built up in your system.

Remember that a human being can go many days without food and survive, but you cannot and should not go any length of time without proper hydration.

What To Eat When Fasting

Since you may not actually go without food during a fast, you need to think about what you eat and not just the number of calories.

Having sugary foods can mean simply spiking your blood sugar and causing you to be hungry, as will eating simple carbohydrates such as white bread and pasta, and starchy foods.

The best foods to eat when observing any type of fast are those high in protein; lean meat choices, such as chicken and fish, or vegetables like broccoli and leafy greens are good, as are eggs.

Protein fills you up and keeps you from feeling hungry and also stabilizes your blood sugar.

Vegetables also provide you the essential nutrients you need throughout the day, as well as fiber to make you feel full and help break down other foods. You might opt for lots of salads, or an omelet to which you add onions, celery, peppers, and spinach.

Since you can and should have lots of hydration during a fast, you might consider making a variety of vegetable soup to have during this time.

Use a low-sodium soup stock or broth and add vegetables high in hydration such as celery, bell peppers, leeks, and onions, as well as cabbage and spinach.

Add in other low-calorie vegetables such as carrots, broccoli, and cauliflower, as your calorie intake allows. Soups like this will fill you up and provide you the nutrition you need during a fast.

Benefits Of Fasting For Detoxifying

When you go long periods of time without any food, your liver is able to clear out more toxins from your system as it doesn't need to keep working to filter the liver you ingest from food.

Drinking lots of water while not eating food helps to break down the foods that are currently in your digestive system, so it's easier for the liver to clear out their toxins.

The bile that is produced by the liver to flush away those toxins can also return to normal and healthy levels, so it doesn't cause damage to your stomach or intestinal tract.

Others who are considering purchasing this book would love to know what you think. If you could spare a few seconds, they would greatly appreciate reading an honest review from you. Simply view the page on Amazon.com.

Chapter 7

Juicing for Detoxifying

Like fasting, juicing can mean not putting new toxins in your body through the foods you eat, and it also helps to flush out those toxins while letting your liver work more effectively.

Juicing refers to either substituting entire meals for certain juice blends, or having those juice blends in addition to meals in order to hydrate your system and give your body the nutrients it needs for a good detox.

If you're thinking of juicing for detoxifying, let's first consider some important points about how to do this safely and effectively.

Homemade Juice

One of the best things you can do to juice safely and to ensure you can detoxify when juicing is to make homemade juice.

As with foods, store-bought juices will have preservatives and other additives that will only add to the toxins in your system. You don't need a fancy or expensive juicer to make homemade juice; you can use a standard household blender and add filtered water to your fruit and vegetable mixes.

This can also allow you to add green tea extract and spices like cinnamon, which are both very good for digestion and detoxifying.

Making homemade juice also allows you endless possibilities as to the flavors and varieties of juices you create, so you don't get bored while juicing to detoxify.

Juice Ingredients

Not all juices are the same when it comes to vitamins, trace minerals, amino acids, and other nutrients needed to flush toxins out of the body and help cleanse the liver. Consider some of the best ingredients you might use for a good juicing cleanse or detox.

Citrus fruits of all varieties contain a high level of natural acids; this may sound harmful, but these acids help to break down toxins and irritants in the digestive system.

Citrus fruits also have a high concentration of vitamin C, which is a building block of your immune system. When your immune system is strong, your liver can function more effectively as a filter for toxins.

Use a variety of citrus fruits in your juices for maximum benefit; squeeze some lemon or lime into a juice blend to reduce their tart flavor and still get their benefits, and don't rely on oranges alone for the citrus fruits you include in your juice blends.

Berries are very high in antioxidants that help to cleanse out the digestive system and build your immunity. These can also cut the flavor of other ingredients you might want to add to your juices.

As with citrus fruits, it's good to use a variety of berries so you get the benefits from all of them, and you might experiment with berries you don't normally have in your everyday diet, such as boysenberries or blackberries.

Grapes are also very high in antioxidants and vitamins, and juicing is a good way to have grapes that you may not like on their own, such as tart green grapes or dark red grapes.

Exotic tropical fruits like mango and papaya are also very high in vitamins and trace minerals and can help to break down toxins in the system, flushing them out.

Mango can be a bit tart and papaya may seem a bit dull on its own, but you can mix these with other fruits for a nice taste, or blending them with filtered water may also create a juice flavor you love.

One thing you don't want to do when making homemade juices for detoxifying is add sugar. Sugar can actually dehydrate you and works as its own toxin.

You can also start to pack on the pounds when you ingest all that sugar, and excess body fat can easily trap toxins, defeating the whole purpose of juicing in the first place!

You might also be careful of straining the juice as you blend it. You may not like the taste and texture of pulp from oranges or ground seeds from certain fruits, but remember that this is where the most fiber and many of the vitamins and antioxidants are contained.

If needed, invest in a high-quality blender that will really grind down these ingredients, and cut the juice with more water to make it palatable, but avoid straining out those added ingredients as much as possible.

You might also consider keeping in the peel or rind of fruits like apples, as this too contains a high amount of fiber and other essential nutrients.

How To Juice For Detoxifying

There are a few different ways you can juice in order to detoxify; one is to use juice instead of meals, as said.

If you're thinking about fasting, juicing can be a better alternative if you've never actually fasted before and don't know how well you'll handle the hunger pains, and especially if you're concerned about your blood sugar levels.

You might start with a light breakfast and lunch of no more than 500 calories combined, and then have two glasses of juice later in the day, one at dinnertime and one before bedtime.

Another way to juice as part of a fast when you're just starting out with this plan is to have a light breakfast and then two glasses of juice during the day for the second day, then have light meals, adding up to no more than 500 calories total for the second day, and then a breakfast and juice schedule again on the third day, and continuing to alternate this way throughout the week.

You might also choose one day during the week to have only juice and few if any solid foods. Pick a day when you will be busy and not as likely to think about food; this might be a Monday when you're busy at the office and won't be as distracted by a growling stomach.

As with fasting, you might still have a small amount of solid food along with your juice; start the day with a glass of juice, then have a banana at 10:00 o'clock in the morning, then juice for lunch, then a handful of nuts at dinnertime, and another glass of juice at night before bedtime.

The sparse calories and protein in the banana and nuts will keep you fueled up but won't overload your system, allowing your liver to work effectively to remove toxins.

It's also good to ensure you don't make yourself sick by going too many days without solid foods, as the body still needs protein in order to regulate blood sugar.

You can add some dark leafy greens and broccoli to your juice mixture to get this protein, if you have a good blender or juicer that will easily mix in these veggies; otherwise, be prepared to have a few slices of lunchmeat, a slice of low-calorie toast with peanut butter, or a small handful of nuts on the days when you decide to juice, so you get this protein and keep yourself healthy.

Another good way to use juicing for detoxifying is if you substitute these healthy juices for other foods and snacks that aren't so healthy.

As said, many foods that are saturated in fats can actually increase the toxins in your system, so cutting them out can allow your body to cleanse those toxins away.

Using juice instead of fatty foods, foods high in sugar, and foods with high levels of other toxins can help the liver to create the enzymes needed for maximum effectiveness.

To use juice instead of such foods, bring some with you to the office and have your juice rather than another snack in the mid-afternoon. At night, have juice rather than chips or other foods you might usually have when watching TV, or before bedtime.

You can even substitute juice for just one meal during the day. This can mean cutting down on the toxins you would otherwise get from your morning bacon or evening steak, and allowing your liver that quick break so it can "catch up" on its detoxifying.

Chapter 8

Detox Drinks and Supplements

Detox drinks and supplements can help to cleanse the liver and flush toxins from your system. Many supplements contain ingredients you can't readily get on your own, and they are mixed in a good ratio that will help the liver to detox quickly and easily.

Other detox drinks can combine certain teas and other simple ingredients that you can find at most health food stores. Note a few suggestions here for the right drinks and supplements and how to use them.

Homemade Drinks

Here is one good homemade liver cleansing drink you can make; start with eight ounces of any citrus juice (freshly squeezed is best), along with the juice of one whole lemon, one clove of garlic, one tablespoon of olive oil, and a piece of ginger about one inch long. Blend this with eight ounces of water.

Another good homemade liver cleanse drink is to combine one large apple including the peel or rind, one stalk of celery, half a piece of ginger, and a bunch of baby carrots.

Broth is also good for liver cleansing if you want a warm juice for cold mornings or for after work. In a stockpot, mix four large potatoes, four large carrots, 2 stalks of celery, three whole beets, two peeled and sliced onions, and a full bulb of garlic. Let simmer for about 30 minutes and then strain out the veggies for a strong, detoxifying broth you can easily reheat when needed.

Teas

Making your own tea blend or using certain roots to steep for tea is also a good way to detox your liver.

Dandelion root is a very strong ingredient used for teas to flush the system and detox the liver, and you might also consider ginger, clove, cinnamon, licorice root, black peppercorns, orange peel, parsley root, juniper berries, burdock root, and horsetail; these last two are available at most health food stores.

Consider steeping some dandelion root and then adding a sprinkle of cinnamon or ginger, or mixing horsetail with your favorite green tea.

You might also mix the sweeter licorice root with a stronger black peppercorn for a very warming and calming tea. A dab of honey in any of these tea mixtures can sweeten the flavor and coat your digestive tract for even more cleansing and better digestion.

Supplements

Liver cleansing supplements can give your body the vital nutrients it needs and the enzymes your liver requires for detoxifying, and they can be a good choice to use if you don't want to make up your own juices, teas, and other beverages for a home detox.

Look for supplements with milk thistle, which is a thorny weed that contains vital nutrients that work to break down toxins in the body. Fennel seed and black walnut shells are also very good ingredients in a supplement to help clean the liver; also, look for ginger root, artichoke leaf, and wormwood, as these are very good ingredients for rebuilding and repairing the organ of the liver.

When you do purchase supplements, be sure you research the brand itself. Some supplements contain more filler than active ingredients, so you want to ensure you're getting a quality variety that contains more of the vital nutrients advertised than powders and gelatin that do nothing.

Also, it's good to note that some supplements work best on an empty stomach, so the liver is better able to absorb their nutrients while it's not breaking down the toxins and harmful ingredients from the food you've just eaten.

Some, however, are better absorbed into the digestive system with food. You may also need to drink a large amount of water when taking a certain supplement, so it can be dissolved thoroughly and work more effectively as it reaches the liver.

There are also supplements that are meant to be used over a specific time period but then no longer. They may activate certain enzymes in the liver to make it work more effectively, but if you keep taking them indefinitely, this may actually cause harm to the liver or cause the supplement to build up in your system.

In all cases, be sure you read the directions carefully and follow the recommendations for how to use a supplement safely and properly so you detox without causing damage.

I hope you have learned something from this book so far and would greatly appreciate it if you could leave an honest review on Amazon.com.

Chapter 9

5-Day Rapid Weight Loss Cleanse

Now that you know a bit more about how clean eating, fasting, and juicing can help to detoxify the liver, you might consider how to combine these, along with your regular eating, for your 5-day rapid weight loss cleanse and detoxifying, in order to cleanse the liver and lose weight from all those toxins your body is holding.

This is because one day of fasting or a day of just drinking juice may not be enough to cleanse the liver and shed unwanted pounds from those nasty toxins in your system.

A 5-day Cleanse

If you follow a 5-day cleanse, you can usually go without much solid food somewhat easily, since it's just for those five days.

Start the first day with a juice breakfast, then a lunch and dinner that follows a clean eating plan, both of which add up to no more than 500 calories combined, then another juice at night. Have a cup of cleansing tea sometime in the day as well.

On the second day, have a clean eating breakfast, juice through the day, and a clean eating dinner, still not ingesting more than 500 calories through the day, and another juice at night.

On your third day, rely on juices alone with only 300 calories of solid food through the day; this might be just a few peanuts and a banana, or an orange and a piece of toast with reduced calorie butter. This is the day your body will really catch up on cleansing and detoxifying. Have two cups of cleansing tea on this day as well, to get rid of those toxins and kick your liver into overdrive.

On the fourth day, have a 250-calorie, clean eating breakfast, then juices throughout the day, and another clean eating dinner of 250 calories at night.

On the fifth day, have juice for breakfast and a clean eating lunch and then a clean eating dinner, and a cleansing tea at night. Have another juice at night if you're feeling hungry before bedtime. As you follow this schedule, switch up the meals you have, as long as they're from a clean eating plan.

Also, it's good to ensure you go at least four hours between having any solid food, so your digestive system can fully break down the foods you eat and your liver doesn't get overwhelmed but can work effectively to rid your body of toxins.

Extending This Cleanse

Once you've followed this five-day cleanse, you might want to repeat it for even more weight loss and more detoxifying. However, give your body a break from your cleansing tea and get some solid food for two days before you try it again.

Have at least 1000 calories from solid food for those two days; 1200 to 1500 calories is even better, to ensure your energy levels don't drop and your blood sugar levels are normal.

When you repeat the five-day cleanse, have different foods the second time than you did the first, so you're not missing out on any nutrients; if you have an orange for a day of your first five-day cleanse, switch to an apple or another fruit, or a cup of berries.

If you didn't have salads on the first round of the cleanse, be sure you have lots of leafy greens during your second cleanse, with healthy olive or avocado oil.

Following A 30-day Cleanse

A 30-day cleanse should never be treated like a five-day cleanse that you just repeat, as this can mean depriving your body of too many calories and nutrients.

Instead, this may involve just some simple, everyday changes that can help your liver to regenerate and work effectively, while also helping you to lose unwanted pounds that are stuck because of those built-up toxins.

There are a few different ways you can follow a month-long cleanse while still being healthy; consider a few tips.

One schedule is to have a light, clean eating breakfast every day and then another very light, clean eating dinner at night, with juice and cleansing tea throughout the day.

Make sure you don't have more than 1000 calories throughout the day, and keep those calories made up mostly of lean protein and vegetable choices rather than breads or anything made with wheat or flour, along with healthy olive or avocado oil, but no fried foods.

This is a very light plan that is good for when you need a simple cleanse but aren't ready to try fasting and juicing alone throughout the day.

Another schedule would be a day-on, day-off rotation of juicing and no more than 500 calories of clean eating foods, followed by a day of clean eating but in whatever portions and calories you choose. The days off will allow your liver to cleanse and regenerate while the days of standard eating will keep your blood sugar levels healthy and ensure you're getting lots of nutrients.

If this is too strict for you, consider following a clean eating plan for six days out of the week, with just one day set aside for juicing and two 250-calorie meals, also of clean eating foods.

During any cleanse, be sure you drink copious amounts of plain water. This will help the digestive system flush out those toxins being broken down by the liver and get them out of your system faster and easier, and ensure easier digestion for the foods you do eat during this time.

Chapter 10

The Top 7 Foods to Eliminate During Your 5-Day Cleanse

When following any program of detoxifying, consider eliminating some foods from your everyday diet altogether, even if they fit in your allotted calories. This can help the cleanse to work more effectively at breaking down and flushing out toxins that you cannot avoid, such as those from protein and fresh fruits and vegetables.

Consider a list of the top 7 foods to eliminate during a cleanse and even in your everyday diet, and how this can be done.

Refined Sugar

Sugar has absolutely no nutritional value whatsoever; it contains no vitamins, trace minerals, amino acids, or anything your body actually needs for nutrition and health. Its sole advantage is to sweeten foods and make them more palatable, and can rightly be considered empty calories.

However, sugar is more than just calories, as it can easily build up in your system and cause your blood glucose levels to spike. In turn, your pancreas works overtime to produce insulin needed to absorb this sugar into your body's cells. All of this can mean hormones and chemicals in your body that are produced just to properly digest this sugar.

Sugar can also make you feel hungry; one of the body's easiest ways to spur the pancreas to produce insulin is to eat.

When your sugar levels are spiked, your body may send signals to your brain, making you think you're hungry so you'll eat and then produce insulin.

When this happens, you may be tempted to reach for foods that are not very healthy and, again, you build up more toxins and impurities in your body.

When reducing sugar in your diet, you may immediately think of baked goods such as cakes and cookies, candy, and soda, and these are certainly the first and most obvious choices to eliminate.

However, you might also check canned and processed items such as soups and salad dressings for their sugar content, and food processing companies often add sugar to these products to make them taste better.

Artificially Colored Foods

Foods often have artificial colors added to them to make them seem more palatable and to appeal to the eyes and not just the taste buds.

These artificial colors, however, are made with chemicals and additives that are toxic to the body and which often cannot be digested and flushed out of the system, but are caught in the liver to be filtered out of the body. Some of these artificial colorings may contain petroleum products and even some known carcinogens.

Foods that are commonly colored with chemicals include breakfast cereal, flavored applesauce, smoked or canned salmon, flavored yogurt, canned salsa and hot sauce, salad dressing, and even pickles. These foods may have colors added to them after they lose their own natural colors in the preparation process.

To avoid ingesting these artificial dyes and colors, consider again the principles of clean eating. Avoid store-bought breakfast cereals and opt for oatmeal instead, and make your own homemade applesauce with raw apples and a touch of cinnamon you blend in a food processor.

Choose plain yogurt and add fresh fruit for flavor, and make your own salsa with fresh tomatoes and peppers.

Vinegar and oil is a much healthier option than bottled salad dressing for many reasons, including the artificial colors added to salad dressing, and if you must have pickles, look for a local farmer's market where you can buy them fresh and without artificial ingredients including dyes.

Note, too, that many canned and jarred fruits and veggies will also have artificial colors added to them, as they also lose their natural coloring when processed and cooked or frozen.

An alternative to these foods is to buy fresh fruits and vegetables in season and then freeze them yourself, or buy canning supplies and store them in mason jars at home versus buying canned varieties at the store.

Meat

While meat can be part of a clean eating plan and contains protein as well as many amino acids your body needs, it's also typically full of fat and toxins that are in an animal's system before slaughter.

Many dairy cows and other such animals are fed a diet full of hormones and growth steroids, in order for farmers to get more meat from each one. These chemicals aren't always destroyed in the food processing and cooking done to get meat to your table, so your body then ingests them.

It can be difficult for many people to eliminate meat from their diet entirely, so consider how you can reduce your consumption in order to give your liver and your digestive system a rest and especially during a cleanse. For example, you might normally have meat at every meal, including bacon or sausage for breakfast, lunchmeat at lunchtime, and then another meat dish at dinnertime.

If so, eliminate meat from one meal every day; have eggs or oatmeal and no meat dish for breakfast, or opt for a big salad with a scoop of hummus for protein and to fill you up at lunchtime.

Learn to cook vegetarian dishes for dinner, such as pasta with a plain tomato sauce and no meat, or stuffed peppers or portabella mushrooms. A vegetable stir-fry can also be very filling, and your store may have vegetarian patties and other meat substitutes that are very tasty.

You might also pick one or two days every week to go without meat of any sort for long-term cleansing. If you're rushed and exhausted every Monday and always look for quick and easy meal ideas anyway, make some meatless vegetable stew ahead of time that you can simply reheat for dinner.

The more meat you can eliminate from your diet altogether, the fewer toxins you'll have build up in your system overall.

Dairy

As with meat, you don't need to actually cut out all dairy when following a clean eating plan or detoxifying, but the more you can eliminate from your diet, the fewer toxins you'll ingest.

Remember that dairy products come from the same source as meat products, so your milk, butter, cream, and yogurt may start out with a lot of growth hormones and steroids that are ingested by the dairy cows.

Chickens may also be fed many hormones and chemicals to make them larger and meatier, and that force them to lay more eggs so that these too may contain many of these chemicals and toxins.

Dairy products also usually contain a number of preservatives that are very toxic to your system and which can build up in the liver, as can the fat in milk, cheese, and other such foodstuffs.

Reducing your intake of these can help your digestive system also work more easily, as it won't be overwhelmed with bothersome lactose.

To reduce dairy in your diet, switch to soy, coconut, almond, or cashew milk rather than dairy milk or cream. Dip your bread in olive oil rather than buttering it at dinnertime, or add a bit of organic honey to your morning toast so you don't need butter. Ranch salad dressing is a favorite for many and has a large percentage of cream or milk, so this is another reason to consider olive oil and vinegar as a salad dressing instead.

If you must have dairy, try to find a local farmer's market where you can buy fresh, organic products that are created without hormones and steroids and which are packaged without preservatives.

As with meat, you might also set some simple goals for how to reduce it, such as going one or two days without dairy completely or switching out just one dairy product, such as butter, for something nondairy.

Unhealthy Oils and Fats

Your body needs certain oils and fats in order to better absorb vitamins and trace minerals from foods; without enough fat in your system, you can even take supplements and still not be getting enough of those healthy nutrients, simply because your body cannot absorb them properly.

However, there are healthy fats and unhealthy fats; unhealthy fats are those that don't break down very easily in your system, so they clog your arteries and surround your organs, including the liver. Not only does this make the liver work harder to function, but that fat will trap toxins in the body.

Fats used in many restaurants for frying are injected with hydrogen to keep them from separating during the transport and storage process; this is why they're called hydrogenated oils.

Vegetable oil, canola oil, and soybean oil are also very heavy and difficult for your body to break down and digest.

Lighter oils like avocado oil and olive oil are healthier for your body and are easy to digest. If you must have fried foods, use a little bit of these oils in a pan and lightly fry the foodstuffs, rather than deep frying.

Use alternatives to vegetable oil when baking, such as soy milk or coconut milk. Remember that many snack foods including chips and pretzels are also fried; avoid these and make your own at home by baking thin slices of potatoes without oil, or opt for air-popped popcorn when you need a crunchy snack.

Alcohol

It should go without saying that you want to reduce or eliminate alcohol when you're trying to detoxify your liver. This can be difficult for some people, but if you have a true addiction to alcohol, you might speak to your doctor about entering a treatment program.

However, if you just enjoy some drinks at night to unwind or like to have your beer on the weekend to kick back, consider how you can reduce your drinking as much as possible.

Switch to virgin versions of drinks, or note days of the week when you won't drink at all. Have drinks with less alcohol such as light beer or white wine, versus mixed drinks and cocktails. You might also limit your alcohol consumption to a certain number of drinks per day or per week, and then not have any more once you reach that limit.

Remember that you're doing this to give your liver a break and to get healthy, so make a good decision about how much you will drink, if any at all, when it comes to alcohol consumption.

Artificial Sweeteners And "Diet" Foods

To avoid sugar and to compensate for cutting out alcohol, you may switch to "diet" foods, including diet soda, low-calorie baked goods, and the like.

However, artificial sweeteners are just chemicals that mimic the taste of sugar, and foodstuffs like diet soda are made with many chemicals that give them flavor and coloring, and that keep them preserved. They may seem like a safe alternative to sweet foods or foods high in fats, but can be just as toxic.

If you want an alternative to sweet foods and beverages, choose recipes that use natural but low-calorie sweeteners like agave, which is a natural fruit syrup, and Stevia, which is extracted from certain plant leaves.

These sweeteners usually have far fewer calories than sugar and may not have the same level of sweetness, but you will ingest fewer additives and chemicals when you cook or bake or make up your own juices with these sweeteners versus relying on commercially produced "diet" foods and beverages.

Don't forget to share your thoughts on this book by leaving a review on Amazon.com. It takes just a few seconds.

Chapter 11

Protecting, Strengthening, and Detoxifying the Lungs and the Blood

The lungs play a very vital role in detoxifying the body, as said; the liver will filter out impurities and harmful irritants that you eat or ingest, whereas the lungs filter out irritants that you breathe in, or that get absorbed into your bloodstream from the skin.

Without strong lungs, those toxins can build up in the body no matter your overall diet and no matter the health of your liver; when you want to detox and especially for better health and weight loss, you need to consider your lungs and blood as well as the liver.

Remember, too, that you won't be able to exercise and work out for weight loss if you have weak lungs and can barely breathe when active!

The lungs and blood are interconnected because the blood flows through parts of the lungs as it makes its way through your circulatory system.

This is to pick up oxygen molecules that are taken in by the lungs and which are then delivered to every cell of the body; the blood also picks up impurities and toxins and then filters these through the lungs, where they are expelled when you exhale.

Oxygen also feeds the blood itself, making it healthier and better able to produce red and white cells needed for a strong immune system.

Protecting The Lungs

Protecting your lungs involves avoiding as many air pollutants as possible; you don't necessarily need to wear a dust mask when out and about every day, but it's good to wear some type of protection when using household cleaners or when painting even a small area of the home.

Quitting smoking is a very obvious choice for protecting the lungs, but you also need to avoid secondhand smoke; insist that guests in your home only smoke outside, and avoid being around coworkers that smoke.

Filters in the home and elsewhere can also keep air clean; a room filter will pull air through a carbon or cloth weave to pick up impurities, and be sure you change the filter in your vacuum cleaner as often as needed so that it can also pull out more dust and dirt from carpeting.

If you notice that your home is quite dusty and you have a hard time keeping up with dust removal, this usually means you need a room air purifier or a better filter for your furnace. You may not realize this, but it's also important that you breathe through your nose and not your mouth. Your nose and nasal passages both have natural air and a mucus linings that are designed to trap pollutants and irritants before they reach the lungs; your mouth and throat don't have these filters.

If you notice that you breathe through your mouth, make a note to stop every few minutes and check your breathing; take long, deep breaths through your nose and do this repeatedly, and your body may then naturally switch to breathing through the nose.

Another area of protecting the lungs and keeping them free from toxins that you may not consider is your car! The exhaust system on your car doesn't just keep it quiet but also pulls fumes and emissions away from the cab of the car to the backside, where they are then expelled.

If your car has a hole in the exhaust pipe, muffler, or any other part of the exhaust system, or if the catalytic converter is not operating efficiently, you may easily be breathing in fumes and very harmful emissions every time you drive.

Keep your car's exhaust running efficiently and in good repair to protect your own lungs as well as the environment around you.

Strengthening The Lungs

Strengthening the lungs so they can better filter out impurities is best done through cardio activities, meaning activities that require you to take in more oxygen.

While lungs are technically an organ, they get stronger the way muscles get stronger; through use. Sitting on the couch won't strengthen your lungs, so you need to get up and get active.

Regular walking, jogging, an aerobics class, biking, swimming, and hiking are all good ways to increase your lung capacity and strengthen those lungs. Other activities like singing and playing a wind instrument also make the lungs stronger.

Breathing exercises also strengthen your lungs; one simple exercise is to sit up straight and then pull air in through your nose for a count of five.

Pull the air all the way down into your belly; you should feel the belly expand as you do. Hold your breath for a count of three and then exhale for another five-count, pushing the air from the belly but through the mouth and not the nose, as this allows for more air to escape.

Repeat this exercise several times, preferably for several minutes. This ensures you bring in lots of fresh air into the lungs and aren't relying on small "gulps" of air that do little to expand your lung capacity.

Detoxifying The Lungs And Blood

Detoxifying the lungs can be done regularly, but you might consider doing this especially if you are a smoker, have recently quit smoking, have been around anyone who smokes, or have been exposed to any type of air pollution or airborne chemical.

Persons who live or work in very dusty or dirty environments should also consider detoxifying the lungs regularly. Consider a few ways to do this.

- Peppermint is a good choice for clearing out the lungs and helping them to expel irritants and pollutants. This is why you may feel your sinuses open up and get cleared out when you breathe in peppermint.

  You can chew raw peppermint leaves or steep them in water for a tea. You can also breathe in the steam, from a safe distance of course, as you steep peppermint leaves and this will open up the lungs and help to clear out toxins and irritants.

- Ginger also contains many compounds and enzymes that help to clear out the lung passages. Ginger tea is a very good choice for cleaning the lungs and strengthening the blood. You can even add raw ginger to your cooking; sprinkle a bit into a juice mix or grate some into a stir-fry.

- Oregano helps to prevent inflammation of the lung tissue and also clears out congestion. Fresh or dried oregano is a favorite choice for any Italian dish when cooking, or you can steep some in water for a fresh tea that can easily clean the lungs. If you don't care for the taste of the tea, safely breathe in the steam of the water after adding some fresh oregano leaves.

- Eucalyptus helps to clear lungs and is often used for those with breathing disorders. It also has antiseptic properties, helping lung tissue to repair and restore on its own.

A few drops of eucalyptus in a humidifier or vaporizer at night can let the lungs clear out while you sleep, and open up your breathing passages for easier breathing at night and less risk of snoring. This is especially good if you have a persistent cough, which usually signals congestion that cannot be cleared out of the sinuses and throat, or a constantly dry throat.

- It may seem like a simple thing, but bringing in lots of houseplants can help to clear the air around you and detoxify your lungs. Plants will pull in carbon dioxide and the irritants it may hold, and then release fresh, clean oxygen.

- You can also clean your lungs by sitting in a hot sauna or steam bath; you can make your own at home by closing the bathroom door and rolling up a towel at the bottom of the door to form a nice deal to the space, and then turning the shower up to the hottest level.

  Sit in that warm steam for several minutes and safely breathe in the warmest vapors possible, to clean the lungs and help coat them with moisture. This is especially good to do during wintertime when lungs dry out; your lungs need their moisture to create the mucus that flushes out toxins.

  Add a good humidifier to your furnace or a room humidifier and use it liberally during cold, dry winter months, or if you notice that you seem to always have a dry and scratchy throat.

- Strong spices in your cooking can also help to clear out the lungs and all the toxins that may be trapped in your breathing passages. Consider any spice that makes your eyes and nose water, as this is part of that cleansing process! Fresh chilies, cayenne pepper, garlic, turmeric, and onions are all good for opening up the breathing.

- Folate or folic acid, one of the B vitamins, is also very good for clearing out the lungs and helping them to get strong in order to rid themselves of toxins.

  Folate is also needed to build healthy red and white blood cells. This folic acid is found in very dark, leafy greens like spinach and kale, as well as lentils and black beans. You can also take a B vitamin supplement if you don't get enough folate in your everyday diet.

- Citrus fruits also bolster the immune system and contain large amounts of vitamin C, which can be used by the lungs to rebuild and repair tissue. Grapefruit and oranges are usually the best choice, and especially during wintertime when cold air may dry out the lungs and cause them to work harder.

  This is also a good time to ensure that you're getting lots of healthy fats in your diet, as these are broken down and used to moisturize and lubricate the organs of the body, including the lungs. Olive oil and avocado oil are always good choices and can be part of your clean eating plan that you follow when cleansing your liver, and these are also very healthy and nourishing to the lungs as well.

Are You ALWAYS Hungry When You Try to Lose Weight?

Discover How to STOP Starving Yourself & Lose Weight FASTER By Eating MORE Food!

For this month only, you can get Kayla's best-selling & most popular book absolutely free – *The Ultimate Guide to Healthy Eating & Losing Weight Without Starving Yourself!*

Get Your FREE Copy Here:

TopFitnessAdvice.com/Book

Discover how you can **start eating MORE food** and see weight loss results faster than ever before. Learn about the 10 most powerful fat-burning foods and how they boost the rate that your body burns fat. And last but not least, finally put an end to your emotional or "bored" eating habits. With this book, readers were able to significantly improve their weight loss results. So, it's highly recommended that you get this book, especially while it's free!

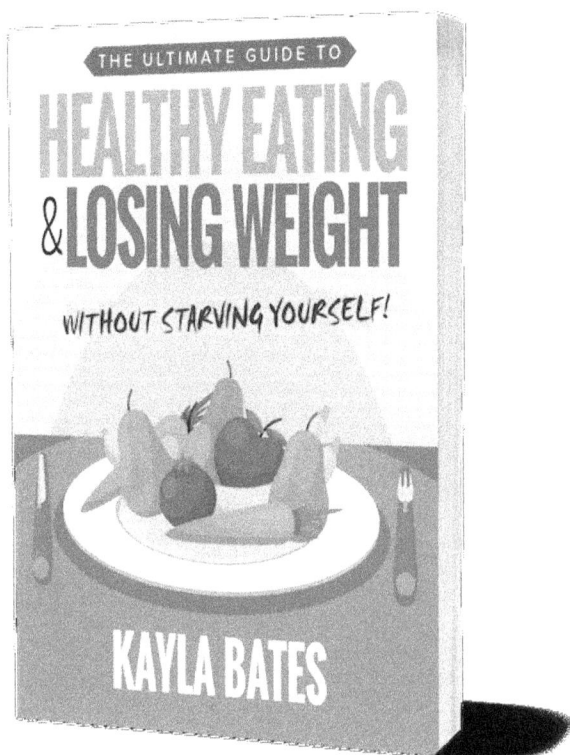

Get Your FREE Copy Here:

TopFitnessAdvice.com/Book

The Most Important Tips for Detoxifying

Let's sum up all you've learned so far with some simple, but the most important, tips for detoxifying your system.

First, protect your liver by ingesting fewer toxins; this means drinking less alcohol and eating fewer foods that trap toxins in your system, including artificial sweeteners, deep-fried foods, and those with artificial colors.

Also, protect your lungs from airborne toxins by avoiding cigarette smoke and car exhaust, and by wearing a mask when exposed to chemicals. Add an air purifier to your home as well.

Don't be afraid to fast or juice to detoxify your liver, but start with something you can manage by allowing yourself 500 calories in a day rather than going without solid food at all.

Choose just one day to do this, and then work up to a longer fast. After this, you can try a 5-day cleanse to remove toxins from the liver and your body overall, and finally lose those unwanted pounds.

Also, even when not following a cleanse, make clean eating a habit; find out where your foods come from and how they're prepared, and put in the work needed to make food from fresh ingredients.

Know the foods that will help your liver to detoxify and that will build strong lungs, and make them part of your everyday diet even if you're not planning an actual detox. This will keep your body strong and keep it as free from harmful toxins as possible, and will make your 5-day cleanse as successful as possible!

Final Words

I would like to thank you for purchasing my book and I hope I have been able to help you and educate you on something new.

If you have enjoyed this book and would like to share your positive thoughts, could you please take 30 seconds of your time to go back and give me a review on my Amazon book page.

I greatly appreciate seeing these reviews because it helps me share my hard work.

You can leave me a review on Amazon.com.

Again, thank you and I wish you all the best!

Enjoying this book?

Check out my other best sellers!

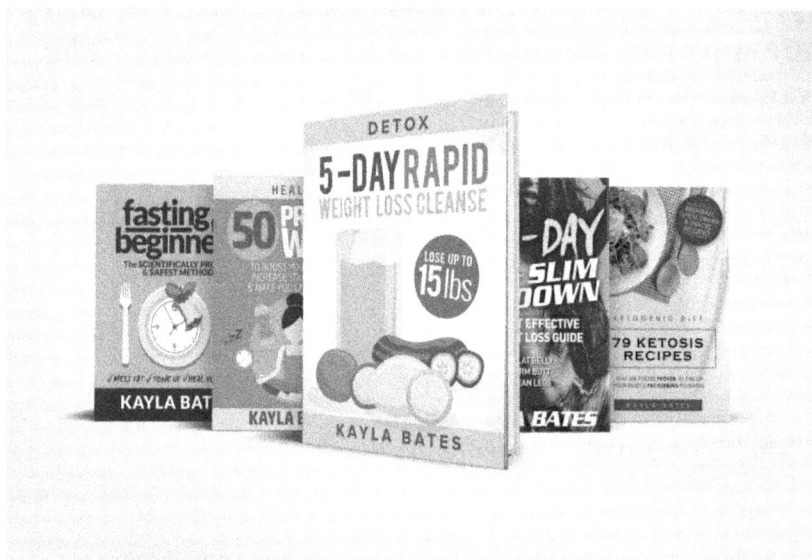

Get your next book on sale here:

TopFitnessAdvice.com/go/Kayla